The Unforgettable Plate

Less is More Cookbook

Suzanne Capizzano

Leaning Rock Press

Leaning Rock Press, LLC
Gales Ferry, CT 06335
leaningrockpress@gmail.com
www.leaningrockpress.com

978-1-950323-58-6, Hardcover
978-1-950323-59-3, Softcover

Library of Congress Control Number: 2021913260

Publisher's Cataloging-In-Publication Data
(Prepared by The Donohue Group, Inc.)

Names: Capizzano, Suzanne, author.
Title: The unforgettable plate : less is more cookbook / Suzanne Capizzano.
Description: Gales Ferry, CT : Leaning Rock Press, [2021]
Identifiers: ISBN 9781950323586 (hardcover) | ISBN 9781950323593 (softcover)
Subjects: LCSH: Cooking, Mediterranean. | Cooking (Natural foods) |
    Vegetarian cooking. | LCGFT: Cookbooks.
Classification: LCC TX725.M35 C36 2021 | DDC 641.591822--dc23

Printed in the United States of America

Dedication

To the beautiful women in my life that have showed me
the art and science of simple healthy foods:
My Nana, Mom and Daughter.

To my supportive husband, **Stephen,**
and the many customers that cheered on the development of
The Unforgettable Plate.

Contents

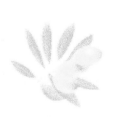

Introduction

These recipes were created from the many events we've featured at Capizzano©
Olive Oils & Vinegars over the years. I hope you enjoy them as much as we do.

In breaking bread together, it is pleasurable to have our senses excited so we
can be more aware of what we are about to experience. You will find that the
flavors presented in this cookbook complement what your palate loves. Food is
medicine and what we choose to put in our bodies is important in our journey
toward health. Less is more. Simple fresh flavors win me over every time.

Enjoy your journey with *The Unforgettable Plate*. Be creative. There are many
delicious options available when pairing the many flavors of high quality Olive
Oils & Vinegars. A sip says it all.

Have fun, be creative, and enjoy.

Per la salute. Suzanne

About Olive oil

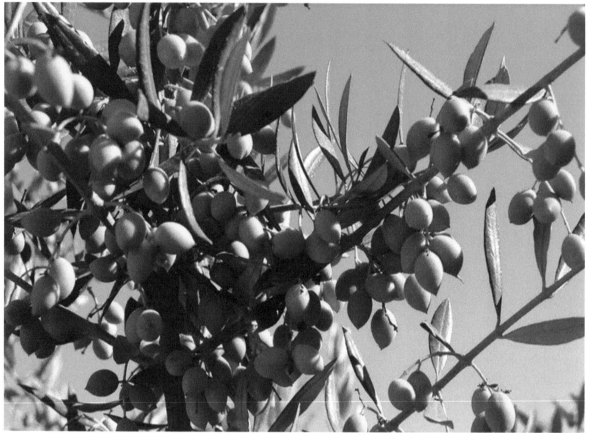

Using extra virgin olive oil in cooking is a celebrated practice all around the world. It is both versatile in its culinary uses and has many different health benefits.

What is Extra Virgin Olive Oil?

Extra virgin olive oil is the highest-quality olive oil, primarily because it is prepared completely through mechanical means without any solvents or chemicals. Unlike many other cooking oils, the oil is kept at a certain temperature throughout the entire crushing process so none of the natural components and nutrients in the oil are compromised. Due to the intensive processing methods, this is the highest quality of olive oil. The taste and aroma should be that of fresh olives, with a pungent, spicy, and slightly bitter taste on the tongue that is quite pleasant.

You can drink extra virgin olive oil in small amounts for its health benefits. When cooking with it, it is important to look at high phenol levels of 320ppm or higher that will keep the olive oil stable longer with temperatures of 420 degrees F.

Extra Virgin Olive Oil Nutrition

In terms of nutrition, extra virgin olive oil provides high levels of vitamin E and vitamin K, as well as phenols, flavanols, lignans, and oleocanthal, many of which are antioxidant in nature. These active compounds and ingredients are what provide so many of the health benefits of this oil. There are 120 calories in a single tablespoon of extra virgin olive oil (EVOO), 100% of which comes from healthy fats. Olive oil is composed of about 73% monounsaturated fat, and approximately 13% saturated fat, as well as 10% of omega-6, and 1% omega-3, which is considered a healthy fat.

Extra Virgin Olive Oil Benefits

The most well-known benefits of extra virgin olive oil include its ability to improve skin health, protect cardiovascular health, stimulate cognition. It may also reduce the risk of certain cancers, regulate diabetes symptoms, and strengthen the immune system.

Skin Care

Cleansing the face and skin with high quality extra virgin olive oil has many benefits. Extra virgin olive oil is packed with antioxidants, such as caffeic acids, squalane, phenol compounds, and flavanols, as well as high levels of vitamin E, all of which can help to reduce oxidative stress and seek out free radicals in the body.

Heart Health

There are a lot of fats in this oil and many of them are monounsaturated fats, which are considered "good" fats for the heart. They can help to reduce overall cholesterol levels, suppress blood pressure, lower your risk of atherosclerosis, heart attacks, and strokes.

Anticancer Properties

A great deal of research has gone into the effects of extra virgin olive oil on cancerous growth in the body. The high antioxidant content in Extra Virgin Olive Oil can seek out free radicals. Oleocanthal is a compoumd in olive oil that is known to rapidly cause cancer cell apoptosis or cancer cell death. There is more information in these articles: *European Journal of Cancer Prevention*, 2004 and Rutgers University, *Ingredient in Olive Oil Looks Promising in the Fight Against Cancer: Oleocanthal kills cancer cells with their own enzymes.* By Ken Branson, 2015.

Obesity

Despite being high in fat, this oil is also linked to improving cholesterol balance, which is one of the major factors behind metabolic syndrome. Regular use of high quality extra virgin olive oil and a healthy lifestyle can help you maintain a healthy weight.

Immune System

Vitamin E is found in measurable levels within olive oil, and this antioxidant compound can do wonders for the immune system. In addition to the other antioxidants, this vitamin can help to lower the strain on your immune system and fight off pathogens and toxins as they accumulate in the body.

Diabetes

High phenol Extra Virgin Olive Oil has benefits to help regulate blood sugar and insulin levels, making it a preferred cooking oil for those with diabetes.

About Balsamic Vinegar

Made from Trebbiano grapes, balsamic vinegar is known for its rich flavor and velvety mouth feel. Balsamic vinegar offers several health benefits and a lot of flavor with a drizzle.

Low in Calories

With balsamic vinegar, a little goes a long way. Use 1 tablespoon or less when adding balsamic vinegar to salad dressings, sauces or even soups. A 1-tablespoon serving of balsamic vinegar has only 10 grams of carbohydrates. The natural sweetness comes from Trebbiano Grapes, there is no sugar added.

Normalizes Blood Pressure

According to a study published in *Medscape General Medicine* in 2006, researchers found that balsamic vinegar reduced the hardening of arteries, also known as atherosclerosis. Because of this, balsamic vinegar also lowers and stabilizes blood pressure levels. Researchers in the study found that those who regularly consumed vinegar exhibited lower systolic blood pressure levels. However, further study on humans is required, as this study was animal-based.

Stabilizes Cholesterol Levels

Low-density lipoprotein cholesterol causes hardened, clogged and blocked arteries. In a 2010 study, published in the *Journal of Nutritional Science and Vitaminology*, researchers found that the polyphenols in balsamic vinegar limited the ability of LDL cholesterol to oxidize. This reduced the amount of damage done by LDL cholesterol on your body's cells.

Regulates Blood Sugar

Perhaps the most important benefit of balsamic vinegar is that it's low on the glycemic index. High glycemic foods, like most factory-processed foods, can result in a sudden spike in your blood sugar. Low glycemic foods can generally keep sugar levels stable for a longer period of time. Keep in mind your portion sizes (1 tablespoon of our 18 year aged balsamic vinegar has 9 grams of sugar with about 36 calories). If you are diabetic, the sweetness from the grapes is a natural fruit sugar.

Breaking the Fast

Breakfast does not have to mean traditional eggs and cereal. I enjoy experimenting with textures, colors, and flavors.

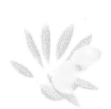

Egg Veggie Bowl

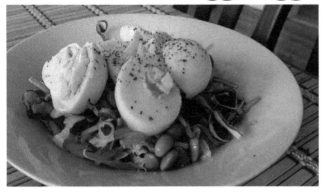

A beautiful presentation, and a feast for the eyes and taste buds.

2 serving

Ingredients:

- 2 boiled eggs, to your preference (soft, medium or hard boiled)
- ¼ cup shredded purple cabbage
- ¼ cup shredded carrots
- ¼ cup edamame, cooked
- Chives, snipped
- 2 La Abuella Olives, chopped
- Capizzano© Herbs de Provence Olive Oil (Options: Basil, Garlic Mushroom & Sage or any robust extra virgin olive oil.)
- Sea Salt to taste
- Fresh ground pepper to taste

Instructions:

1. Hard boil eggs to desired preference, shell and slice in half.

2. In shallow bowl, add each item in sections or mix together. Shredded cabbage, carrots and edamame putting the halved eggs on top,.

3. Add a couple of chopped olives, then sprinkle the snipped chives all around.

4. Drizzle Capizzano© Herbs de Provence Olive Oill on top of the Egg and Veggies. Season with some sea salt and pepper. Enjoy with some toast and honey butter.

Egg and Avocado Boat

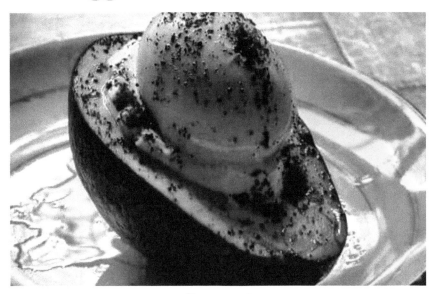

Serves 2

Ingredients:

- 1 avocado, cut in half, pitted.
- 4 - 6 tablespoons of cottage cheese or plain Greek yogurt or ricotta cheese.
- 2 boiled eggs (soft is my preference) shelled.
- 4 tablespoons Capizzano$^{©}$ Extra Virgin Olive Oil
- Sea Salt
- Za'atar spice

Instructions:

1. Add cottage cheese or plain Greek yogurt in the hollow to pitted avocado.

2. Add the boiled shelled egg on top.

3. Sprinkle your sea salt and or Za'atar spice on top.

4. Drizzle a generous amount of your favorite extra virgin olive oil on top.

5. Enjoy healthy fats, good protein and tons of flavor.

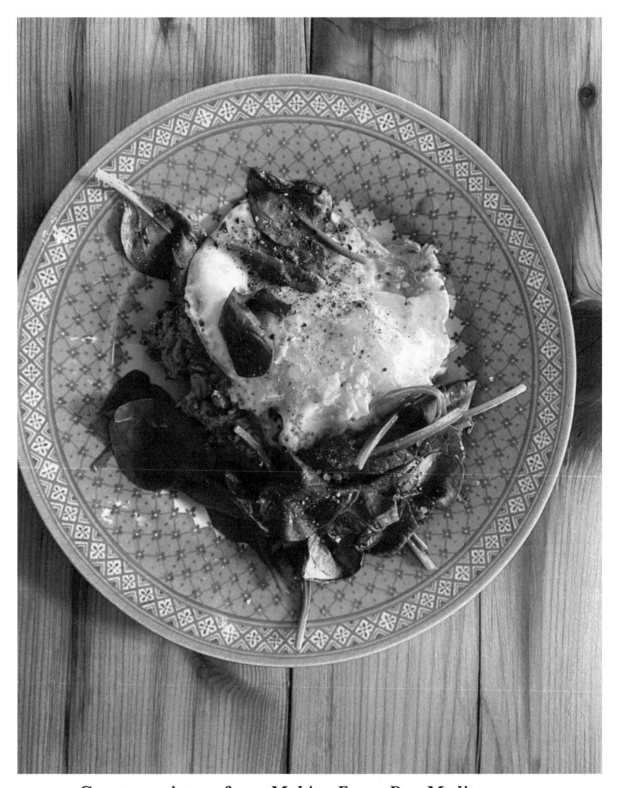

Courtesy picture from _Making Every Day Mediterranean_

Farro Egg Spinach Bowl

This can be a meal filled with dense nutrients that will keep you satisfied for a long time. Drizzle with your favorite Capizzano© Olive Oil to complement this meal.

Ingredients:

- Egg, over easy or scrambled
- Farro, prepared as package directed
- Baby Spinach
- Basil Infused Olive Oil (or your choice of Capizzano© Olive Oil)
- Korean red pepper flakes
- Sea Salt to taste
- Fresh ground pepper to taste

Instructions:

1. Prepare egg as desired. Both types of cooked eggs are delicious.

2. Prepare farro ahead of time.

3. Sauté baby spinach until just wilted in a pan with a little robust extra virgin olive oil, season to taste with sea salt and Korean red pepper flakes.

4. Place cooked farro in bowl.

5. Add wilted seasoned spinach and top with the egg.

6. Drizzle a little Basil Infused Olive on top.

7. Season to taste with a bit of sea salt and pepper.

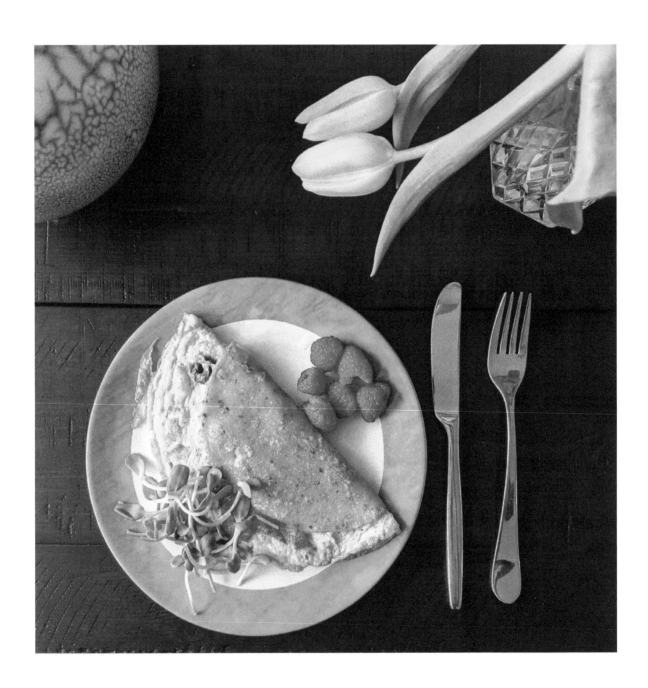

Tortillas Anytime

Our favorite meal: Tortillas.
For breakfast, lunch, or dinner.

1 serving

Ingredients:

- 2 eggs
- Diced Kalamata olives
- feta or mozzarella chees
- Capizzano© Pesto
- Organic corn tortillas
- Your favorite Capizzano© Olive Oil

Instructions:

1. Heat a large non stick fry pan on high.

2. Add 1 TB of a robust Capizzano© Extra Virgin Olive Oil to the pan.

3. Scramble 2 eggs , spreading thinly like a crepe.

4. Sprinkle diced Kalamata olives and feta or mozzarella cheese over eggs.

5. Spread Capizzano© Pesto on an organic corn tortilla.

6. Press pesto side into egg. Flip over together. Cook 1-2 minutes on tortilla side and fold in half.

7. Serve with microgreens and berries.

Extra Note:

For a spicy topping, whisk Capizzano© Baklouti Chile Pepper Fused Olive Oil and freshly ground Black Pepper in with a touch of sour cream. Drizzle on top of the tortilla.

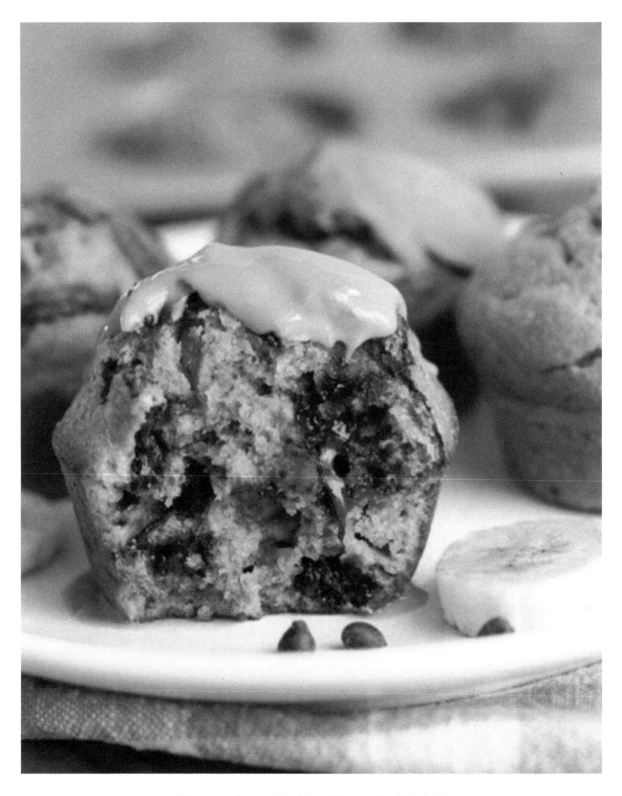

(Picture from *Making Thyme for Health.*)

Flourless Peanut Butter Banana Muffins

I love these muffins. They are moist and delicious for a treat during the day with tea or coffee. The original recipe from *Making Thyme for Health* is slightly modified.

Yield: 12 Muffins

Ingredients:

- 2 ripe bananas (approx. 1 cup mashed)
- 2 eggs
- 1/4 cup unsweetened oat milk
- 1/3 cup pure maple syrup
- 1/2 cup creamy peanut butter
- 1 teaspoon vanilla extract
- 2 and 1/4 cup quick cooking rolled oats
- 1 teaspoon cinnamon
- 1 teaspoon baking powder
- 1/2 teaspoon baking soda
- 1/4 teaspoon salt
- 1/3 cup dark mini chocolate chips

Instructions:

1. Preheat oven to 375 degrees and grease a muffin tin. Set aside.

2. Combine all of the ingredients, except the chocolate chips, in a blender; adding wet ingredients first. Blend for 30 seconds, or until a smooth batter forms.

3. Add mini chocolate chips and gently stir into mixture.

4. Baking time is about 18 minutes, check with a toothpick to make sure the middle is cooked. Let cool completely before serving.

5. Mix 3 tablespoons creamy peanut butter with a teaspoon of Dark Chocolate Aged Balsamic Vinegar and drizzle it on top before serving. The muffins will last 4 days in a covered container.

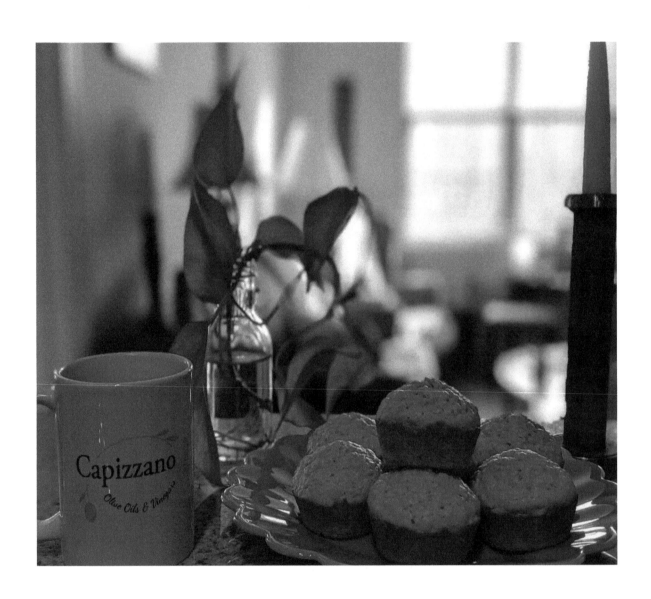

Oatmeal Muffins, using Capizzano© EVOO!

This is a modified version from Yellow Farmhouse in Stonington, CT. I used our Arbequina Mild Intensity EVOO, providing more healthy fats instead of butter.

Ingredients

- 1 cup All-Purpose Flour
- 1 cup quick oats
- 1/2 cup brown sugar
- 1/2 teaspoon salt
- 1 tablespoon baking powder
- 1 cup almond milk
- a little less than a 1/4 cup Mild Intensity Extra Virgin Olive Oil (or 5 tablespoons melted unsalted butter)
- 2 large eggs
- 1 teaspoon vanilla extract

Instructions:

1. Mix all ingredients together.

2. Oven 375 degrees for about 18 minutes.

3. Do the toothpick test at 15 minutes. When toothpick comes out clean, they are done.

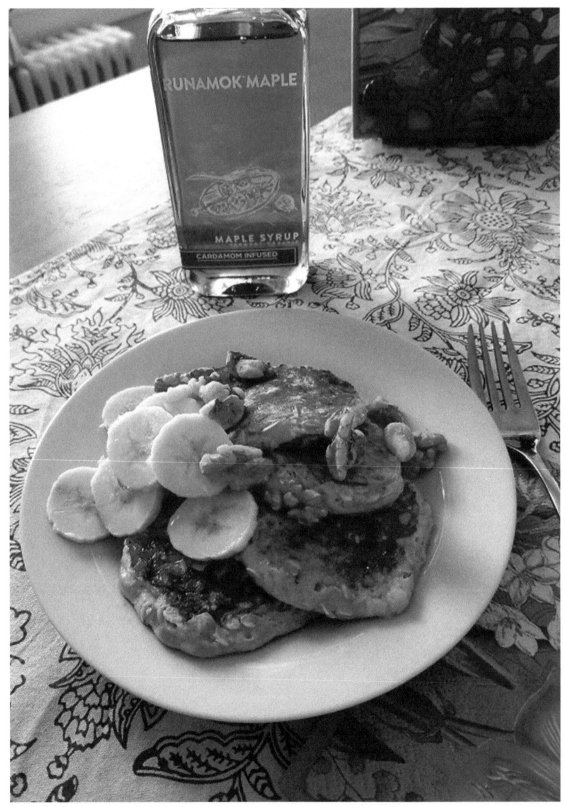

Banana Oat Flourless Pancakes

My daughter, Amanda, made these for me during my visit. They are so easy to make, and I feel good about eating them. Since I try to remove gluten from my diet, I have also used organic oat bran by Bob's Red Mill; this works as well as the oatmeal. Enjoy them!

Makes 8 Pancakes

Ingredients

- 2 Banana, large, very ripe
- 1 cup quick cooking Gluten Free oatmeal
- 3 eggs
- 2 level teaspoon baking soda
- 1 tablespoon pure vanilla extract
- Sea salt, a dash
- 1 heaping tablespoon ground flaxseed meal
- Capizzano© Butter Infused Olive Oil
- Maple Aged Balsamic
- real maple syrup

Instructions

1. Blend bananas, eggs, oatmeal, baking soda, vanilla extract, salt and flaxseed meal together on high for a minute or two until smooth.
2. Preheat skillet or large pan on medium high and grease with coconut oil or butter.
3. Cook about 2 minutes on each side. You will see bubbles at edges of pancake when its time to flip it over.
4. Whisk Capizzano© Butter Infused Olive Oil and Maple Aged Balsamic with a bit of real maple syrup.
5. Drizzle on top of pancakes before serving (this decreased the sugar and saturated fats).

Notes:

Of course you can use real butter and maple syrup, either way they are delicious and gluten free.

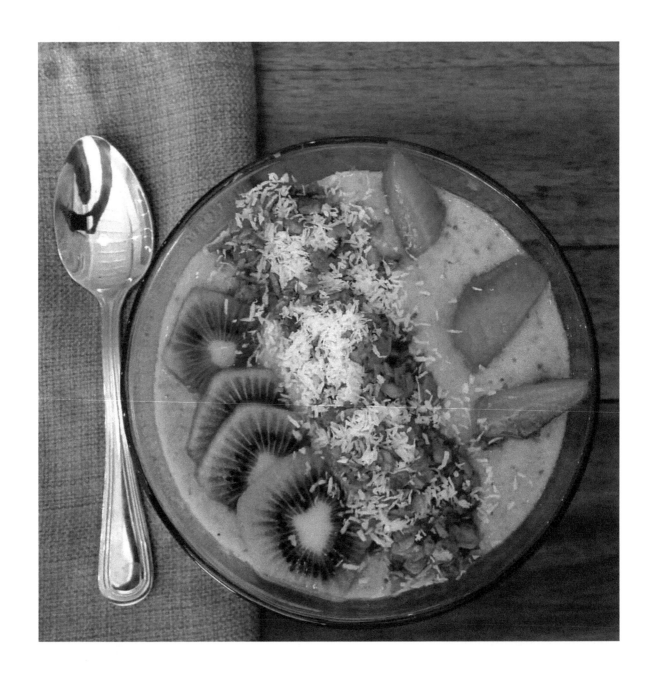

Smoothie Bowl

Ingredients:

- Spinach, small handful
- Avocado, pitted
- banana
- mango
- 2 TBS Persian Lime or Lemon Olive Oil
- coconut water
- Strawberries, halved
- Kiwi, sliced
- Granola or crushed nuts and seeds
- Shredded coconut

Instructions:

1. Blend these ingredients together on high; it should be thick and smooth.

2. Mix in a little Coconut Aged Balsamic Vinegar with the fruit. Let stand 10 minutes.

3. Put the smoothie base in the bowl. Add fruit on top. Add granola and shredded coconut on top. Enjoy

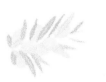

The Main Event

Featuring many dishes with vegetables, legumes, and fish. Each dish is simple to make, wonderful to look at and satisfying to you tastebuds.

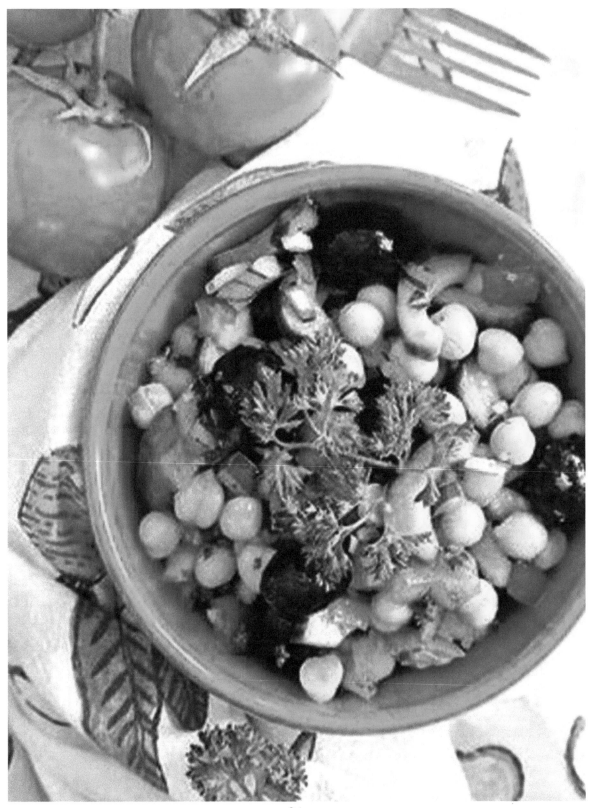

Olive, Tomato and Chickpea Salad

Oh my goodness!

This salad is refreshing, flavorful and, with Capizzano© olives and olive oil, this salad shines. It is great alone or with your favorite lean protein.

Yield: 4 servings

Ingredients:

- 1 pint cherry tomatoes, halved
- 2 small crisp cucumber, washed and cubed
- 1/2 cup Capizzano© Garlic Stuffed or La Abuela olives, halved
- 3-4 tablespoons of Capizzano© Medium or Robust Premium extra virgin olive oil
- 1/4 cup chickpeas, drained and rinsed
- juice of 1/2 of a lemon
- 1/2 teaspoon dried oregano
- sea salt and black pepper to taste

Instructions:

1. Toss all ingredients together in a small mixing bowl.

2. For best flavor, serve at room temperature or chill.

Black Rice and Vegetable - Warm Salad

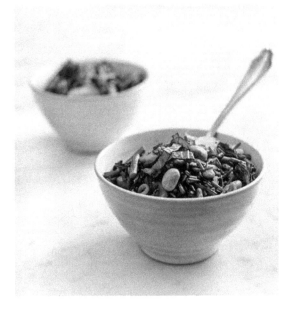

4 servings

Texture and flavor define this salad. You can use any of your favorite vegetables; just make sure you cook them to a tender crunch to complement the black rice.

Ingredients:

- 1 - 1/2 cup of vegetables (your choice of Brussel sprouts, broccoli, string beans, carrots, lima beans or edamame.)
- 2 ½ cups diced butternut squash
- 4 tablespoons Capizzano© Butternut Squash Seed Oil or any Extra Virgin Olive Oil, divided
- ¼ teaspoon salt, plus more to taste
- ¾ teaspoon chili powder
- 1 cup Capizzano© Italian Venere (Black) Rice
- 1 cup legumes/beans, cook as instructed on package first.
  *Optional: use 1 can kidney or cannellini beans, drain and rinse.
- Juice of 1 lime
- 4 ounces regular or vegan feta, crumbled or diced
- Pepper to taste

Instructions:

1. Preheat oven to 425 degrees.

2. Cook dry bean according to package directions. *Or use the canned beans, drained and rinsed well.

3. Toss the vegetables and butternut squash with 2 tablespoons of the Butternut Squash Seed Oil or olive oil, along with the salt and chili powder.

4. Spread the seasoned veggies in a thin layer over a parchment-lined baking sheet and bake for 25-35 minutes, until golden, tossing halfway through.

5. While the veggies are baking, cook wild rice according to package instructions, then drain off any excess water.

6. In a large bowl, combine the cooked wild rice with the roasted vegetables and squash.

7. Add the legumes/beans, pepper, and lime juice, along with the remaining 2 tablespoon Butternut Squash Seed Oil or olive oil.

8. Taste and adjust seasoning (salt and pepper) if necessary.

9. Divide into 4 portions and serve warm or chilled. I like it warm.

10. Drizzle a little of your favorite Capizzano© Olive Oil on top upon serving.

Kiwi Edamame Rice Salad

If the Kiwis are just ripened, you can keep the skins on; just scrub them well and cut the ends off. I eat my kiwi this way. If they are too ripe it is best to take the skins off. This recipe originated from Nadia Bakes. I modified it to incorporate Capizzano© Olive Oils & Vinegars.

Salad Ingredients:

- Small, sweet onion, diced up
- 2 crunchy cucumbers, quartered.
- 8 – 10 kiwis, washed and scrubbed well, cut off ends; then keeping skin on, cut into quarters.
- Feta cheese, break apart into small pieces, about ¾ of a cup.
- Fresh dill, snipped to garnish top
- Sesame seeds, black and white to sprinkle on top
- 2 cups, frozen edamame, cooked
- 4 cups of Capizzano© black rice, cooked
- 1 cup cottage cheese
- 1 cup red cabbage, finely chopped
- 1 lemon zest
- A good handful of fresh parsley, chopped

Dressing Ingredients:

- 1 lemon freshly squeezed.
- 1 cup of your favorite Capizzano Olive Oil (Lemon or Basil Olive Oil is great in this recipe)
- 1/3 cup local honey
- 2 tablespoons fresh grated ginger

Instructions:

1. Mix dressing ingredients together; Set aside.

2. Put the warm rice on the bottom of large serving bowl.

3. Add warm edamame, cold cottage cheese, red cabbage, lemon zest and fresh parsley.

4. Pour dressing on top and gently fold in together.

5. Garnish with dill and sesame seeds.

Date Almond Salad

**This is great with fresh baked bread
or part of a meal with fish and black rice.**

Ingredients:

- 8 pitted dates, sliced partially in half
- 1 cup Almonds, slivered
- 2 cups Arugula
- Parmesan cheese, shaved
- Capizzano© Extra Virgin Olive Oil (Medium or Robust Intensity)
- Capizzano©Mission Fig Aged Balsamic Vinegar
- Sea Salt

Instructions:

1. Arrange the fresh arugula leaves on a flat serving platter.
2. Put almond slivers inside partially cut dates, and place the dates with almonds on top of the arugula.
3. Garnish the arugula and dates with shaved parmesan cheese and some slivered almonds.
4. Whisk the Extra Virgin Olive Oil, Fig Balsamic Vinegar and sea salt together; drizzle on top of the salad, making sure to get some in the dates. Use a 2:1 ratio with olive oil to vinegar. You can add more or less of each depending on your taste.
5. Drizzle Olive oil dressing over the salad, being sure to get some in the dates.

Options:

Lemon Fused Olive Oil with Sicilian Lemon Aged Balsamic are great also. There are many different flavor pairing you can try with this salad.

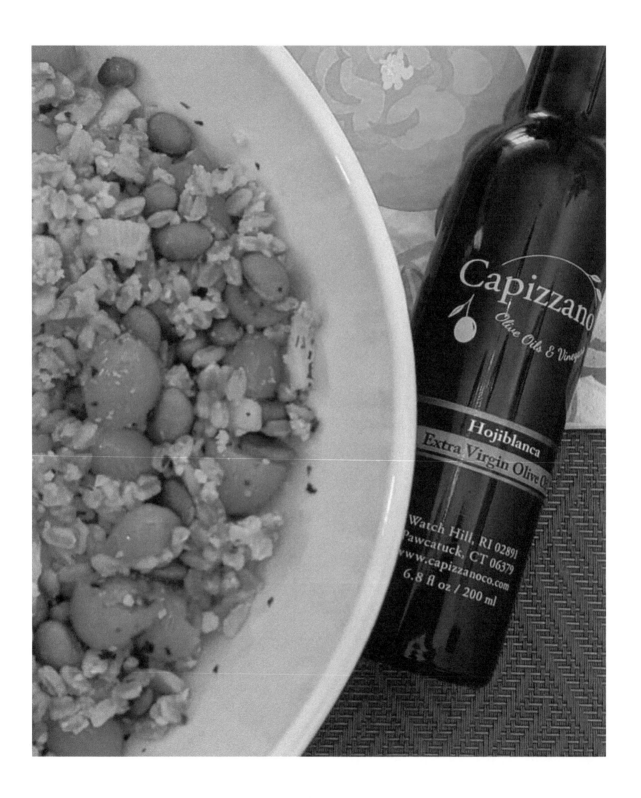

Italian Farro Tomato Salad

This is a customer favorite salad. We sold it at a farmer's market and it got rave reviews. It is a mixture of different textures, with added protein, fiber, and mouth-watering goodness. Add your favorite vegetables from the summer or fall harvest and enjoy with any Capizzano© Olive Oil.

Ingredients:

- 1 package of Farro from Italy, cook as directed
- 2 cups of grape tomatoes, washed, cut in half
- ¼ cup of a robust extra virgin olive oil (I used Picual EVOO)
- Sea Salt 1/8 teaspoon
- 1 onion sliced in quarters, thinly
- 3 heaping teaspoons of minced garlic
- Basil dry herb about 1 teaspoon
- Edamame, cooked and drained
- String beans, cut up, steamed until just tender
- OPTIONAL: Parmesan Cheese, fresh grated, on top to serve.

Instructions:

1. Soak the farro in fresh water for about 20 minutes. Rinse and cook it as the package directs until tender crunchy not mushy.

2. While Farro is cooking, add grape tomatoes, onions and the minced garlic to a shallow pan with extra virgin olive oil, salt and herbs. On medium heat warm up until onions are translucent.

3. Put drained Farro in large bowl, add olive oil and tomato mix to the Farro.

4. Add cooked string beans and the edamame; Toss together.

Optional:

- Add freshly grated parmesan cheese.
- Garnish with snipped fresh basil leaves and drizzle more extra virgin olive oil on top when serving..
- Serve immediately on top of tender greens.

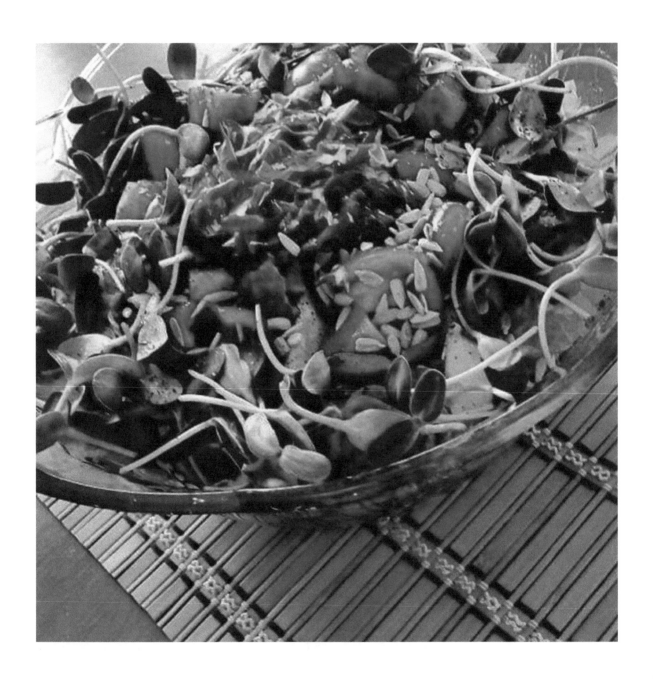

Suzanne's Salad

Serves 12 people.

This is my favorite salad. I love the colors that pop with each fresh vegetable tossed in it. Any combination of Capizzano© Olive Oil and Vinegars will complement it.

Ingredients:

- 1 bag small Organic Crunchy Cucumbers, washed, cut up in cubes
- 2 pints Grape tomatoes, washed and halved
- 1/2 of a medium head of purple cabbage, thinly sliced and thinly cut up
- 4 Scallions, thinly sliced
- 2 cups Kale leaves, stems removed
- 2 cans Organic, no salt chickpeas or kidney beans
- a small handful of fresh microgreens
- Garnish with raw sunflower seeds

Instructions:

1. Put cut up ingredients in large salad bowl, Toss together.

2. Add mixed EVOO dressing on top; toss together to coat the vegetables.

3. Serve immediately.

Dressing:

- 1/3 cup Koroneiki Extra Virgin Olive Oil (high phenolic level)
- 1/4 cup Sicilian Lemon Aged Balsamic Vinegar
- 1 Tablespoon Fennel Seed, crushed in a mortar & pestle
- 1 Tablespoon Basil, dried herb
- Newport Pure Sea Salt, 1 Teaspoon or to taste.
- Whisk together very well, pour on top of the salad ingredients.

Options:

- Wild Dill Olive Oil and Grapefruit Balsamic is tasty!

Salad Love Time

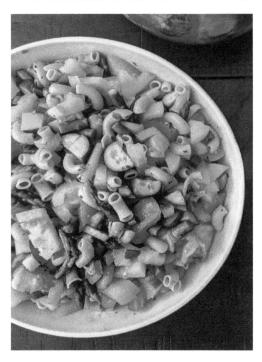

Ingredients:

- Your choice of pasta, cook as package directs
- Crispy cucumbers, cut up
- Heirloom tomatoes, two different color tomatoes, cut up
- Scallions, diced
- Asparagus, tender tips and stems, steamed
- Korean pepper flakes
- Sea salt
- Capizzano© Garlic Infused Olive Oil

Instructions:

1. Cook pasta as directed, drain.

2. Place pasta in bowl with other cut up vegetables and ingredients.

3. Generously pour the Garlic Infused Olive oil over salad

4. Toss and serve.

Scrumptious Beef and Cabbage Soup

A clean and nutrient packed soup with lots of flavor!

Ingredients:

- 1 lb. grass fed ground beef
- 4 tablespoons of a robust Extra Virgin Olive Oil (I used Picual from Spain)
- ½ small heads of red and green cabbage; sliced and diced
- 4 sliced carrots
- large handful of fresh string beans, cut up in small sections
- 1 box or jar of beef bone broth
- 1 can of Tuttarosa crushed tomatoes
- ¼ - ½ teaspoon oregano,
- ¼ - ½ teaspoon sweet basil,
- ¼ - ½ teaspoon garlic powder,
- ¼ - ½ teaspoon celery salt,
- ¼ - ½ teaspoon turmeric
- ground pepper to taste
- small handful of fresh snipped cilantro
- drizzle of Basil Infused Olive Oil.

Instructions:

1. Saute the ground beef until browned.

2. Add 4 TBS of Extra Virgin Olive Oil

3. Add cabbage, carrots, and string beans. Sauté for a few minutes.

4. Add beef bone broth and crushed tomatoes; Stir and simmer until vegetables are crunchy tender.

6. Add the oregano, sweet basil, garlic, celery salt, turmeric and ground pepper to soup

7. Just before serving add the cilantro to the pot.

8. Serve with a drizzle of Basil Infused Olive Oil.

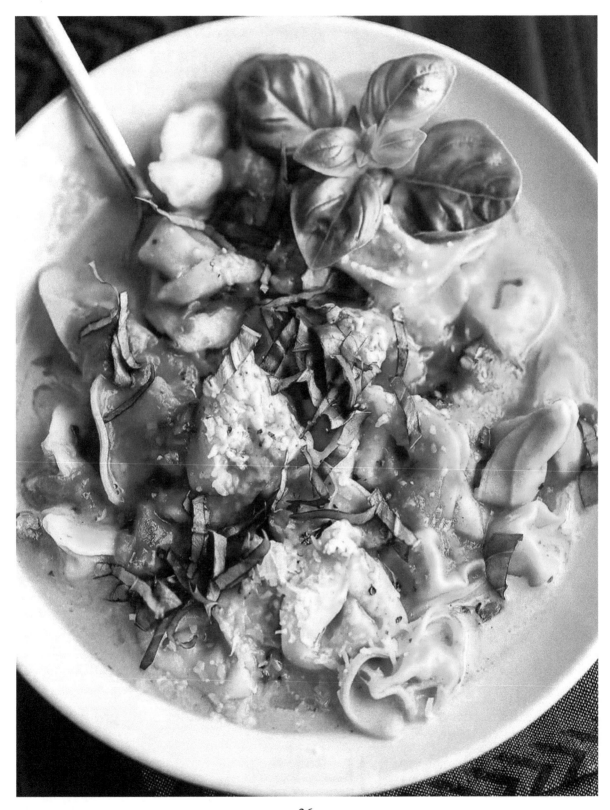

Capizzano© Tortellini Spinach Soup

Our absolute favorite when we are entertaining guests.
This soup has it all.

Ingredients:

- 5 garlic cloves, sliced thinly
- 2 sweet onions, diced
- 4 tablespoon **Capizzano©** Extra Virgin Olive Oil, (I used our 'Melgarejo' Picual EVOO)
- A Pinch of Oregano (fresh or dried)
- 1/2 teaspoon Sea Salt from Sardegna Italy
- Organic Bone, Chicken, or vegetable broth, 32 ounces
- "Pomodoro e Basilico" or other spagetti sauce 23.9 ounces
- Tortellini, frozen, 1 package
- 2 cups or large handful fresh, non GMO spinach

Instructions:

1. Boil water and prepare tortellini per directions on package. Keep tortellini on the firmer side before adding to sauce. I cook just under 5 minutes. Cook and Drain. Set aside.

2. Sauté in large pot the garlic and onions with EVOO, oregano and sea salt for about 4 minutes on medium heat.

3. Pour organic chicken bone broth and "Pomodoro e Basilico" sauce in sauteed mixture. Keep heat on medium - low, let simmer for 10 minutes. Stir. Lower heat.

4. Add the cooked and drained tortellini to sauce gently stir.

5. Just before serving add the fresh baby spinach to the pot. Stir gently.

6. Serve immediately with a Drizzle of Capizzano© Basil Infused Olive Oil on top of soup.

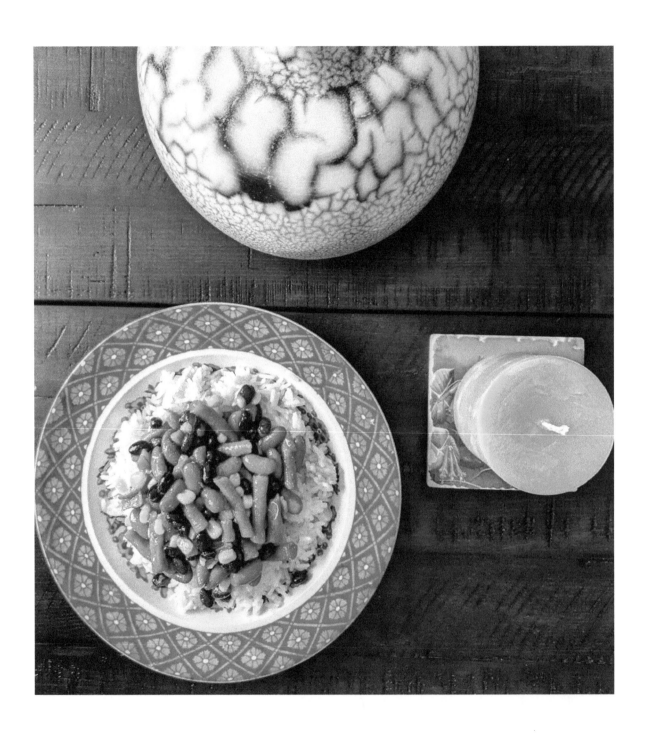

Suzanne's Rice and Beans

My go to meal is this rice and bean recipe.
I often make a double batch to last me for a few days.

Ingredients:

- 1/4 cup Garlic Infused Olive Oil
- 1 teaspoon Sea Salt
- 1 tablespoon cumin,
- 1 tablespoon sweet paprika,
- 1 teaspoon oregano,
- 1 teaspoon onion powder
- 1 teaspoon garlic granules
- 2 cups Jasmine, Basmati or Brown Rice
- 1 can organic black beans, drained and rinsed
- 1 can organic kidney beans, drained and rinsed
- 1 small bag of organic string beans, cut up, and steamed.
- 1 cup corn fresh or frozen, steamed.
- 1 can of organic diced tomatoes.

Instructions:

1. Cook Rice as directed and keep warm; set aside.

2. Mix together the Garlic Infused Olive Oil, Sea Salt, cumin, sweet paprika, oregano, onion powder and garlic granules in a glass cup; whisk together.

3. In a large saucepan, mix together the bean and vegetables; simmer on low for 10 - 15 minutes.

4. Place the cooked rice on a serving dish. Add bean mixture on top of rice.

5. Enjoy with a fresh salad and toasted naan bread.

Root Vegetable Casserole Dish

**This dish is the definition of comfort food that is good for you.
It warms the soul.**

Serves 6 to 8

I have added root vegetables to this cassoulet along with a few mushrooms. Feel free to add vegetables or greens of your choosing. The heartier the better. Cut the baby root vegetables in half to extend their reach. If the turnips come with nice tops, wash well, cut them up and add them to the cassoulet.

Ingredients:

- 4½ cups cooked borlotti beans or kidney beans
- Capizzano© robust extra virgin olive oil, generous amount
- 10 pearl onions
- Kosher salt
- Freshly ground black pepper
- 1 cup diced carrots or 12 baby carrots
- 1 cup diced turnip or 9 baby turnips with greens washed and chopped
- 1 cup dice parsnip
- 1 cup diced celery
- 6 medium shiitake mushrooms, cap only, thinly sliced
- 3 large white oyster mushrooms, cap only, thinly sliced
- ¼ cup Pomodoro Basil tomato sauce
- Seasoned breadcrumbs

Instructions:

1. Preheat the oven to 350 degrees.

2. Place the drained beans in a large bowl.

3. Heat a large sauté pan over medium high heat. Add the extra virgin olive oil (EVOO) of your choice then add the pearl onions and brown. Season with salt and pepper. Add to beans in bowl.

4. Repeat with the carrots, turnips, parsnip and celery root, cooking in batches until they are golden and seasoning as you go. Reduce the heat if the pan gets too hot and starts to burn.

5. Add the mushrooms to the cooked root vegetables and cook until the juices are almost dry. Add to the beans. If you have turnips greens cook them now in a little EVOO until wilted and add them to the bowl.

6. Add the tomato puree to the pan and stir until it bubbles. Add 1 cup of water, stir well and pour over the vegetables in the bowl.

7. Transfer the beans and vegetables to a large 4-quart baking dish or casserole dish. Top with the breadcrumbs.

8. Bake until the casserole is bubbling, and the breadcrumbs are golden, about 1 hour. If the breadcrumbs brown too quickly cover lightly with a sheet of aluminum foil. DO NOT seal or the breadcrumbs will get soggy.

Healthy Salmon and Salad Dinner

Serves 2

My brother, Scott, gave me this recipe a long time ago. I added our olive oil and balsamic vinegar, and it was a different meal; the flavors of the fresh seasonal olive oil and aged 18 year balsamic made it all come together.

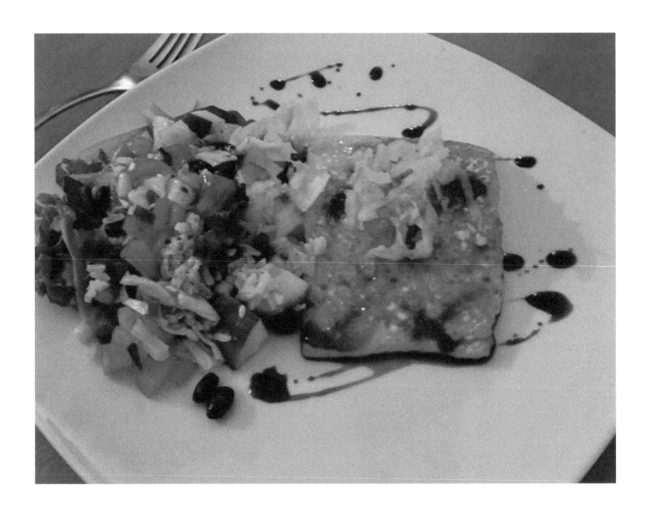

Salad Ingredients:

- 1 head of Iceberg or romaine lettuce, cut in small chunks
- 1 can black beans, drained and rinsed
- 1/2 cup Feta crumbs, Mozzarella Pearls or Cheddar cubed
- 1/2 cup corn, fresh from the cob or frozen (cook briefly and cool)
- 1 cup tomatoes, cubed
- small handful of parsley or cilantro, snipped
- 2 Salmon fillets; baked or grilled as desired
- Garlic Infused Olive Oil; for the salmon fillets
- Salt and pepper to taste

Dressing Ingredients:

- Capizzano© Extra Virgin Olive Oil
- 1/2 cup traditional Aged 18-year Balsamic Vinegar
- Sea Salt
- Fresh ground peppercorns

Instructions

1. Whisk Dressing ingredients together; Set aside

2. Marinade salmon fillets in Garlic Infused Olive Oil, sea salt and pepper.

3. Grill or bake the salmon fillets to your preferred time. I use an air fryer for 7 minutes at 350 degrees for 2 fillets.

4. Serve the salmon and salad on the plate. Drizzle the salmon with the dressing mix right before serving.

Pasta and Extra Virgin Olive Oil

We have been fortunate to have a few food bloggers from Oregon and Canada feature our olive oils and vinegars. This is one of their featured pasta dishes made with a plant-based protein, gluten free pasta. It is a satisfying meal with your choice Capizzano© Olive Oil and Vinegar. I make this salad often during the warm months with fresh tomatoes and cucumber.

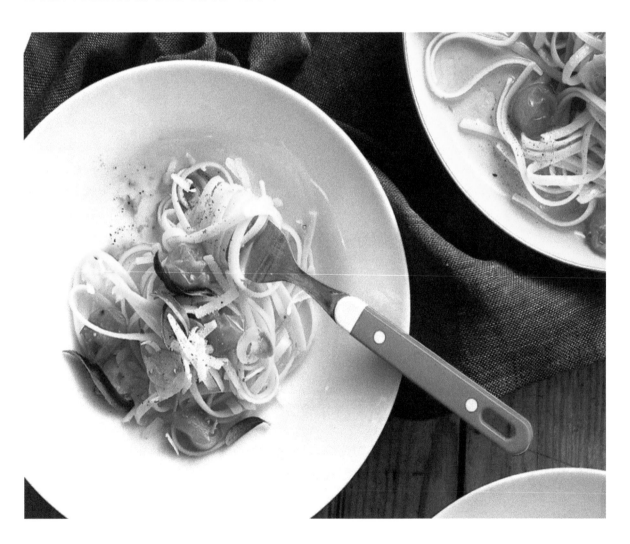

Ingredients:

- 1-pound PrimoGran spaghetti or traghetti, cook as directed
- 2 tablespoons salt (for the boiling water)
- 1/4 cup Capizzano© Robust or Medium Intensity Extra-Virgin Olive Oil
- 8 garlic cloves, minced
- 1/2 teaspoon red pepper flakes
- 2 teaspoons fresh squeezed lemon juice
- 3 tablespoons, finely chopped, fresh parsley
- 2 tablespoons snipped fresh basil and oregano
- 1 cup cherry tomatoes, cut in half

Instructions:

1. Cook pasta as directed.

2. Sauté tomatoes and minced garlic for few minutes on medium heat in 1 tablespoon Extra Virgin Olive Oil. Add premium sea salt to taste.

3. Whisk the remaining Extra Virgin Olive Oil with the lemon juice and salt.

4. Drizzle the olive oil mix on top of the pasta.

5. Garnish pasta with the fresh herbs. Toss well. Enjoy.

Peas of Mind Soup

Celebrate spring with this healthy vegetable soup. This recipe is from *StonyBrook WholeHearted Foods* from the Finger Lakes in New York, using their Butternut Squash Seed Oil. We featured this at a spring tasting event with a special Finger Lakes Riesling and it was a big success. Enjoy with a slice of pumpernickel or sourdough bread.

Ingredients:

- 1 medium onion, roughly chopped
- 2 cloves garlic, minced
- 3 tablespoons Capizzano© Butternut Squash Seed Oil
- 1/2 cup broccoli florets
- 1 10-ounce package of frozen peas
- 1/2 pound potatoes, roughly diced
- 1 small bunch parsley, stems removed
- 1 bunch watercress or 1/2 cup chopped spinach
- 1 cup chopped green cabbage
- 6 cups chicken bone broth or vegetable broth
- 2 teaspoons Sea Shakes Original Seasoning
- 1 teaspoon lemon juice
- handful of basil leaves, cut into strips

Instructions:

1. In a large saucepan, sauté onion and garlic in butternut squash seed oil on medium heat until onions are translucent and softened; about 5 minutes.

2. Add all remaining vegetables and chicken stock; bring to a boil.

3. Lower heat to simmer and cook until vegetables are tender; about 20 minutes.

3. Puree the cooked vegetables in a food processor or blender.

4. Season with Sea Shakes Seasoning and lemon juice to taste.

5. To serve, garnish with basil leaves and drizzle with Butternut Squash Seed Oil. Garnish with shredded purple cabbage and some roasted pepitas from Stony Brook Whole Hearted Foods©.

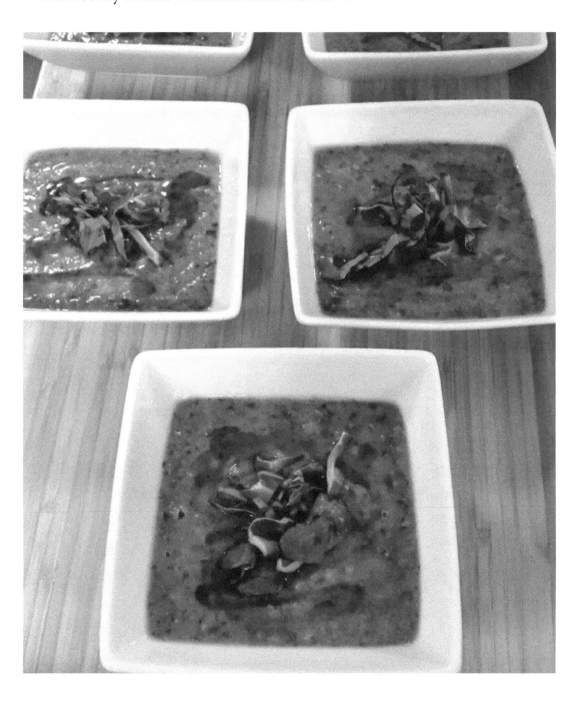

Honey Ginger Sesame Miso Noodle Bowl

Serves 4

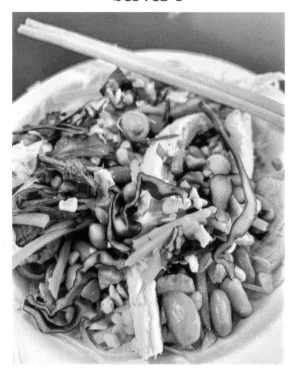

Ingredients for the Honey Ginger Balsamic Miso Dressing:

- 2 tablespoon white or yellow miso
- 1 tablespoon Capizzano Sicilian Lemon White Balsamic
- 2 tablespoons Capizzano Honey Ginger White Balsamic
- 1 tablespoons Capizzano Garlic Olive Oil
- 1 tablespoon Capizzano UP Extra Virgin Olive Oil of choice
- 2 tablespoon Capizzano Roasted Sesame Oil
- 1 teaspoon minced ginger, optional

Dressing Instructions:

Whisk all the dressing ingredients in a medium sized bowl or mason jar until, smooth, thickened and slightly emulsified or place in blender and process until smooth.

Bowl Ingredients:

- 4 chicken breasts or tofu
- 1 package Soba Noodles
- 1cup Edamame, par boil frozen, drain
- 1 cup Carrots, grated
- 1 cup Cucumber, diced
- 1/4 cup Scallions, chopped
- 1 cup Red Cabbage, shredded
- 1/4 cup Chopped Roasted Peanuts or Pistachios,
- Cilantro, snipped; use to garnish the top.

Instructions:

1. **Chicken:** Slow poach 4 chicken breasts in slow cooker or boil in large pot with water or broth, salt and pepper – remove from pot, slice chicken when tender.

2. **Soba Noodles:** add to boiling water in a medium pot, turn heat to medium and add soba noodles, soak until tender (about 5 mins) then drain and rinse in cool water.

3. Serve noodles in a bowl and top with chicken, edamame, carrots, cucumbers, scallions, red cabbage and Honey Ginger Sesame Miso Sauce.

4. Garnish with roasted nuts and cilantro. Season to taste as needed.

Note: Use tofu for a vegetarian/vegan plate.

Modified recipe from *Veronica Foods.*

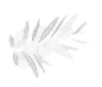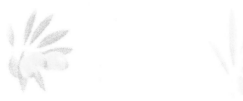

Sweet Indulgence

When I am in the mood for a sweet indulgence, it
needs to satisfy me and come in small portions.
These easy ideas do the trick.

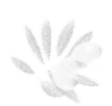

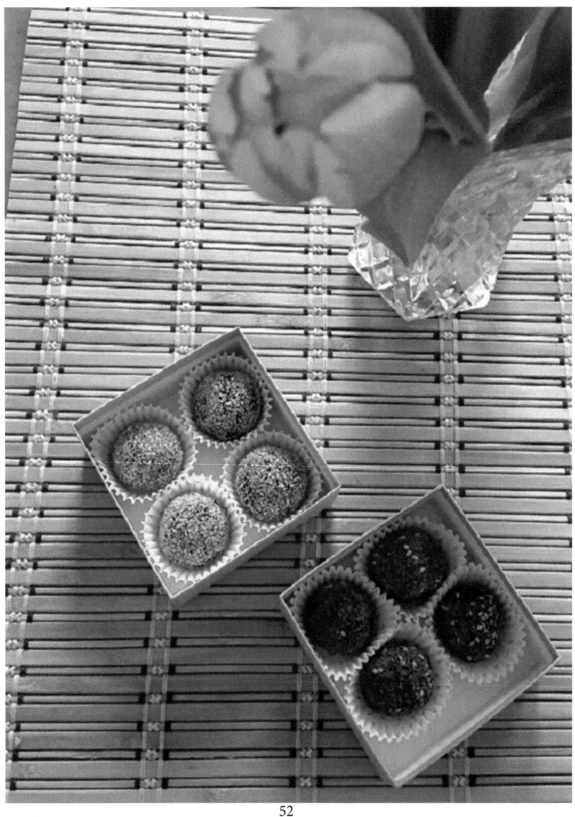

Savoy Truffles

Ingredients:

- 2 cups raw almonds, finely ground in a processor
- ½ chocolate or carob powder
- ½ teaspoon sea salt (optional)
- 1 cup shredded unsweetened coconut
- ½ cup raw honey
- 2 tablespoons of Capizzano© Coconut Aged Balsamic Vinegar
- 2 tablespoons of a robust intensity Capizzano© Extra Virgin Olive Oil

Options:

- 2 tablespoons Blood Orange Fused Olive Oil is delicious too!

Instruction:

1. In a mixing bowl, combine the almonds, chocolate or carob powder, salt and shredded coconut and mix very well.

2. Add the honey Coconut Aged Balsamic Vinegar and Capizzano© Olive Oil

3. Mix until a dough like consistency is reached.

4. Using your hands roll the mixture into small balls, cover with shredded coconut if desired.

5. Cover and chill before serving.

Orange Olive Oil Dreamsicle Cake

Compliments of *Veronica Foods*,
Modified for Capizzano© Olive Oils and Vinegars.

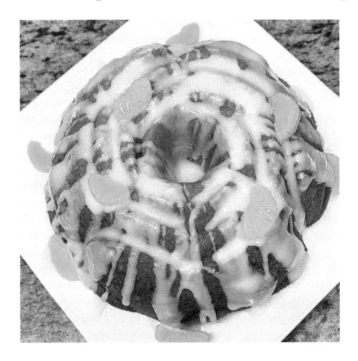

Ingredients:

- 5 large eggs, at room temperature
- 1 cup sugar
- 3 tablespoon finely grated orange zest
- 1 cup Orange Fused Olive Oil
- 2 cups cake flour
- 1 1/4 teaspoons baking powder
- 1 teaspoon vanilla extract
- 1 teaspoon fine sea salt

Orange Cream Cheese Glaze (optional)

- 4 oz. Vegan cream cheese (or dairy cream cheese) at room temperature
- 1 teaspoon grated orange rind
- 1 tablespoon Orange Fused Olive Oil
- 1 teaspoon vanilla extract
- 1/3 cup sifted powdered sugar
- 2 tablespoons original unsweetened oatmilk (room temperature)

Instructions:

For the Cake:

1. Preheat the oven to 325 degrees and grease a 10-cup Bundt pan with coconut oil or butter, dredge with flour.

2. In a bowl, using a hand held electric mixer, beat the eggs with the sugar, vanilla extract, and orange zest at medium-high speed until smooth.

3. Gradually beat in the orange olive oil until creamy, about 2 minutes.

4. In a small bowl, whisk the cake flour with the baking powder and salt.

5. Add the dry ingredients to the egg mixture in 3 batches, beating on medium speed between additions.

6. Scrape the batter into the prepared pan.

7. Bake in the center of the oven until a toothpick inserted in the center of the cake comes out clean; about 1 hour.

8. Let cool in the pan for 15 minutes,

9. Then invert onto a rack and remove from pan.

10. Let the cake cool completely before glazing, cutting into slices, and serving.

For the Glaze:

1. Beat the cream cheese, orange rind, olive oil, and vanilla extract at medium speed of a mixer until smooth.

2. Add sugar and milk and beat at low speed until well-blended.

3. Pour over cooled cake and serve.

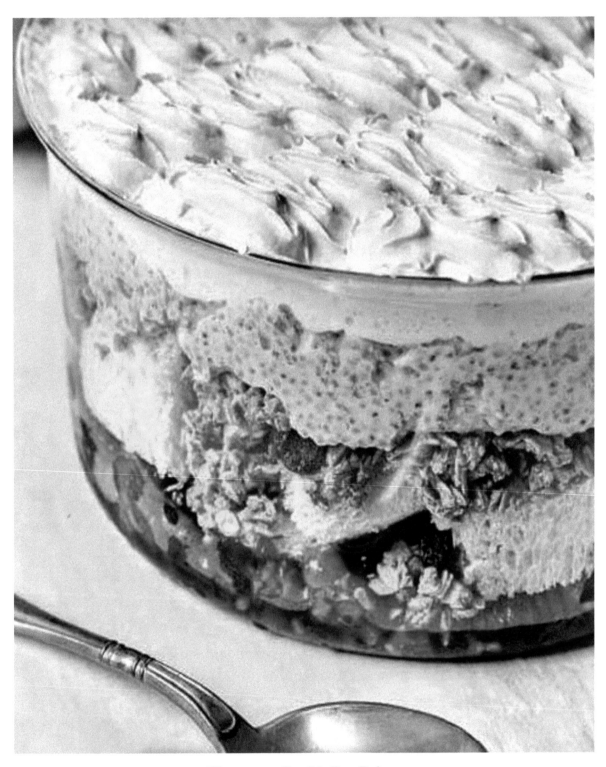

Photo credit, *Nadiya Bakes.*
Capizzano© Olive Oils & Vinegars modified original recipe.

Just Right Berry Trifle

Serves about 8

Ingredients:

- 2 cups Greek yogurt,
- 1/2 cup Chia seeds,
- 3 tablespoonful of Capizzano© Lemon Fused Olive Oil,
- 4 tablespoons of local raw honey, divided
- 2 cups Granola, your choice
- Angel Food cake, cut up (about half of the cake)
- 3 cups fresh Berries,
- 2 tablespoons of Capizzano© Sicilian Lemon Aged Balsamic Vinegar
- 2 tablespoons of local honey.
- Coconut Whipped Cream. Or regular whipped cream.

Instructions:

1. Mix together until smooth the yogurt, Chia seeds, Capizzano© Lemon Fused Olive Oil and 2 tablespoons honey; set aside.

2. Mix the fresh Berries, Capizzano© Sicilian Lemon Aged Balsamic Vinegar and remaining 2 tablespoons of local honey; Save juice to drizzle on top.

3. Layer the ingredients into a large clear bowl as follows:
   - a) Berry Mixture
   - c) Angel Food cake, torn into small chunks
   - d) Granola, spoon at edges of glass bowl.
   - e) Yogurt/chia mixture

4. Top with Coconut Whipped Cream.

5. Finally, spoon remaining berry mix and juice on top.

Note: layers may be repeated if desired.

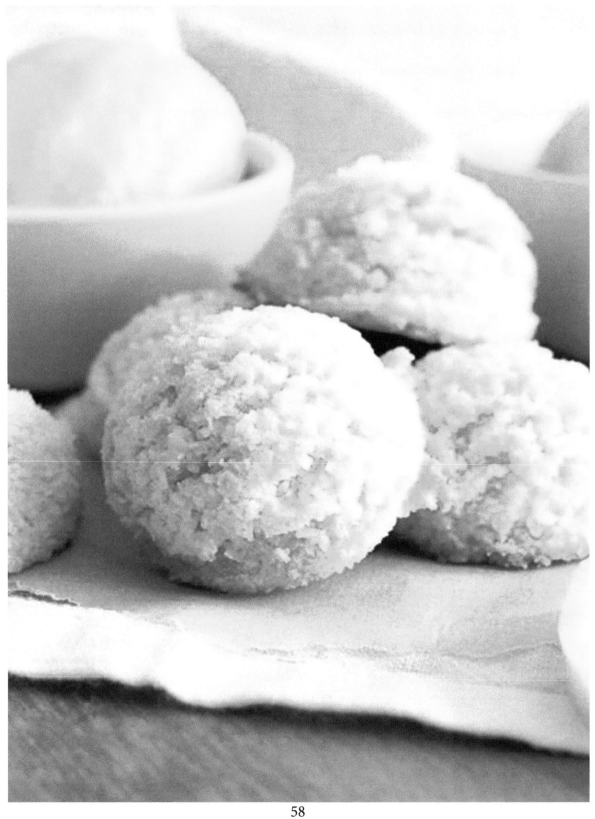

Lemon Macaroons
with Lemon Fused Olive Oil.

Ingredients:

- 6 cups shredded unsweetened coconut
- 14 oz coconut condensed milk (original condensed milk works well also)
- ¾ cup I used Gluten Free almond super fine flour
- 2 tablespoons Capizzano© Lemon Fused Olive Oil (Persian Lime or Mandarin Fused Olive Oil is another option)
- 2 Lemons (the juice and zest of both lemons)

Instructions:

1. Preheat oven to 350 degrees.

2. In large bowl, stir together the coconut, condensed coconut milk, Lemon Olive Oil, the lemon juice, the lemon zest and flour.

3. Drop by 2 TBS rounded scoops onto a parchment paper lined baking cookie sheet.

4. Bake about 15 minutes or until coconut starts to brown slightly.

5. Let cool completely before storing in a container.

Option:

To garnish the cooled lemon macaroons, heat dark chocolate and drizzle a little bit zig zagged on top of the macaroon.

Fruit and Cream Dessert

Ingredients:

- 2 cups fresh berries (raspberries, blueberries and strawberries)
- 1 cup peaches, ripe, pitted and cubed
- 2 tablespoons of raw honey.
- ¼ cup + 3 Tablespoons, divided, Peach Aged Balsamic Vinegar
- Whipping Cream

Instruction:

1. Whisk together the Peach Vinegar and honey.

2. Pour over the fruit and toss gently.

3. Add 3 tablespoons of Peach Aged Balsamic Vinegar into whip cream while whipping into stiff peaks.

4. Top fruit with flavored whipped cream upon serving.

Strawberry Balsamic Vinegar & Ice Cream

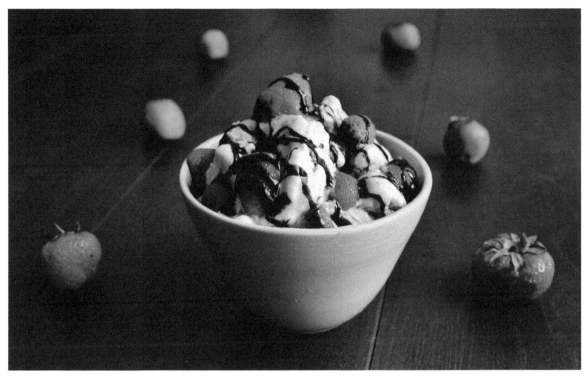

Instructions:

1. Scoop two small balls of vanilla ice cream in a small dish.

2. Add fresh strawberries on top.

3. Drizzle with Capizzano© Strawberry Balsamic Vinegar then serve.

Options:

You can also use blueberries with Blueberry Aged Balsamic Vinegar or raspberries with Raspberry Aged Balsamic Vinegar.

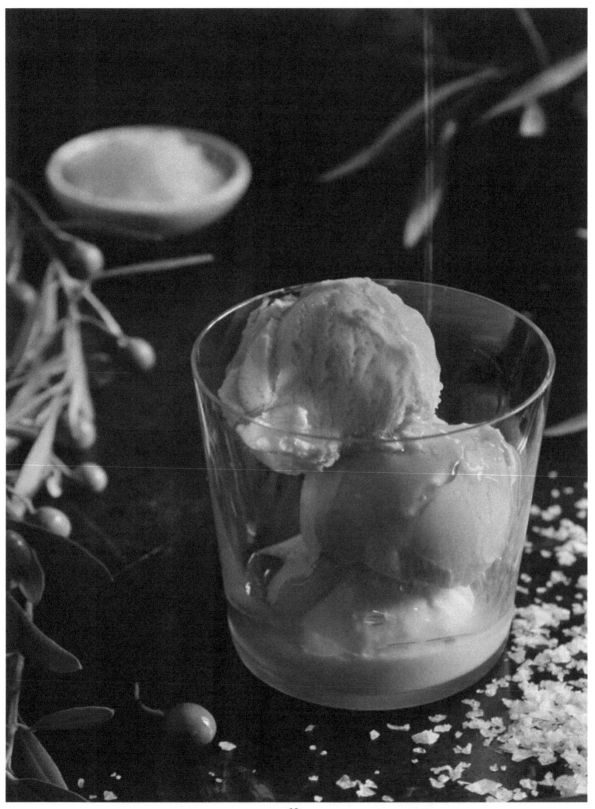

Olive Oil & Ice Cream

A gourmet dessert that is simple to make.
Your guest will be surprised that you used olive oil!

Ingredients:

- Vanilla Ice Cream
- Blood Orange Fused Olive Oil
- Sea salt
- shaved dark chocolate

Instructions:

1. Scoop two small balls of premium vanilla ice cream in a small dish.

2. Drizzle Blood Orange Fused Olive Oil on top.

3. Garnish with a pinch of sea salt and shaved dark chocolate.

Pick Me Up

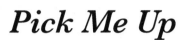

When I need a snack, I like to choose a healthy pick me up.
These are scrumptious and easy to put together.

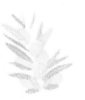

Orange Fennel Salad

Enjoy this refreshing salad alone as a pick me up or with fish.

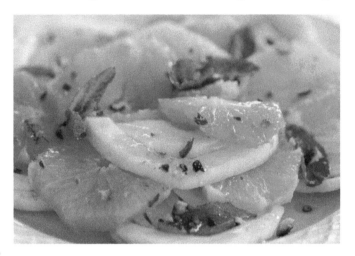

Ingredients

- 3 – 4 Naval Oranges or Cara Cara Oranges, peel well, cut flesh of the oranges in round medallions.
- 1 small bulb of fennel, very thinly shredded.
- Small handful or scallions, snipped thinly.
- Blood Orange Fused Olive Oil
- Sicilian Lemon Aged Balsamic Vinegar
- Sea Salt to taste
- Fresh ground pepper to taste.

Instructions

1. Arrange the oranges and fennel on a shallow bowl or platter and sprinkle the scallions on top.

3. Whisk the dressing ingredients together.

4. Drizzle the dressing generously on top of the oranges, fennel and scallions.

Vertical Caprese Salad
Serves 2

There are many great options with the vast varieties of Olive Oils and Vinegars. Use Garlic, Basil, Herbs de Provence Infused Olive Oil or any seasonal crushed Extra Virgin Olive Oil in this salad. Enjoy the summer harvest!

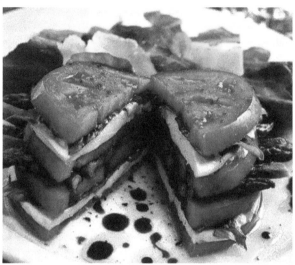

Ingredients

- 3 Heirloom tomatoes, washed, sliced thickly
- 4 round Mozzarella slices
- Small bunch of asparagus, tender tops, steam until tender crunchy.
- Small handful of fresh basil leaves, snipped.
- Capizzano© Robust Intensity Extra Virgin Olive Oil
- Aged Balsamic Vinegar
- Sea salt
- Ground pepper

Instructions

1. Layer and stack the tomato, mozzarella cheese, tomato, asparagus, tomato, mozzarella cheese, basil leaves, and tomato.

2. Pour your choice Capizzano© Olive Oil and Aged Balsamic Vinegar on top, season to taste with sea salt and pepper.

Pineapple – Cucumber Gazpacho

Serves 4 - 6

Ingredients:

- 4 cups chopped peeled cucumber (1 ½ crunchy English cucumber)
- 4 cups chopped ripe pineapple (1 large pineapple)
- 1 cup fresh pineapple juice
- 1 small jalapeno pepper, seeded and diced
- 1 green onion, white and green parts, chopped
- 1 tablespoon lime juice
- 2 teaspoons premium sea salt
- 1 small handful cilantro leaves, washed (save a few leaves for garnish)
- 3 tablespoons Capizzano© Lemon or Persian Lime Olive Oil
- 2 tablespoons Capizzano© Pineapple or Sicilian Lemon Aged Balsamic Vinegar

Optional:

Garnish with 1 handful of finely chopped macadamia or pistachio nuts.

Instructions:

1. In blender, add 3 cups each of the cucumber and pineapple, the pineapple juice, jalapeno, green onion, lime juice, and salt. Blend until smooth.

2. Add the remaining 1 cup of cucumbers, 1 cup of pineapple, handful of cilantro, 1 ½ tablespoons of the Olive Oil and 1 tablespoon of the Aged Balsamic Vinegar; pulse the blender a few times so that the gazpacho remains chunky.

3. Taste for seasoning.

4. Put in refrigerator to chill.

5. Before serving, add the finely chopped nuts on top.

6. Whisk the remaining Olive Oil and Aged Balsamic Vinegar together to drizzle on top of the gazpacho.

7. Garnish with cilantro leaves for color.

Black-eyed Pea Dip

A fun, flavorful dip that is versatile and tasty on your charcuterie or as a main salad with your choice of protein like fish or chicken. The flavors are incredible, with a robust intensity Capizzano© Extra Virgin Olive Oil. There are many options to create with this recipe. Great with freshly baked bread, tortilla chips or a lean protein like salmon.

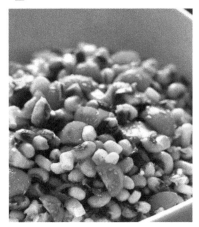

Ingredients:

- 15 oz canned, drained and rinsed, black eye peas (Goya Brand)
- 2 cloves garlic, crushed or minced
- 3 tablespoons fresh lime or lemon juice (from about 1 1/2 limes/lemons)
- 4 tablespoons robust extra virgin olive (such as Picual, Coratina or Koroniki)
- 1 teaspoon cumin
- pinch crushed red pepper flakes
- 1/2 teaspoon kosher salt
- 1 cup cooked corn, cooled (fresh or frozen, thawed)
- ½ cup cooked edamame, cooled
- 1 cup cherry tomatoes, halved
- 1/4 cup minced red onion, finely diced
- 1/4 cup cilantro, chopped
- 1 jalapeño, seeded and diced (optional)
- 1 medium avocado, diced

Instructions:

1. Rinse and drain the black-eyed peas in a colander.

2. In a large bowl, combine the garlic, lime or lemon juice, oil, cumin, crushed red pepper, and salt and mix well.

3. Add the black-eyed peas, corn, tomato, red onion, jalapeno if using and cilantro; mix well and refrigerate at least 20 minutes.

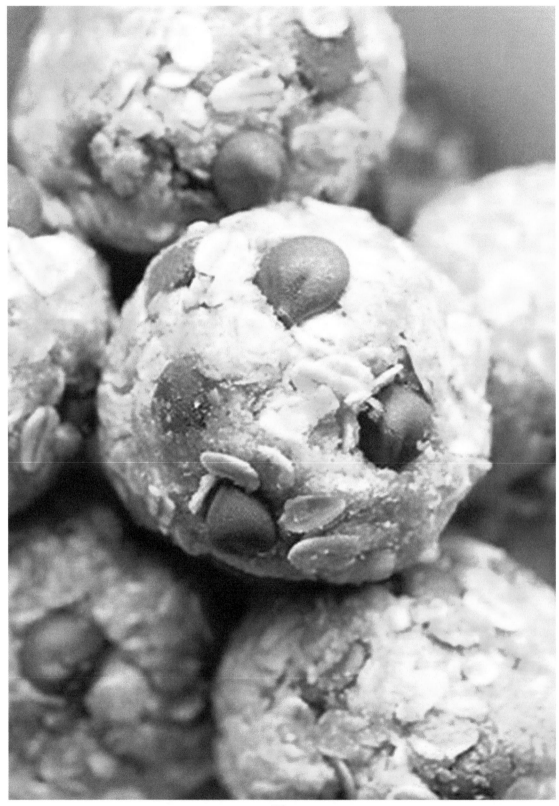

Protein Bites

Ingredients

- 2 cups almonds, coarsely ground in food processor
- ½ teaspoon sea salt
- 1 cup raisins, currants or mini dark chocolate chips
- ½ cup sunflower seeds
- ½ cup raw honey or maple syrup
- 1 cup nut butter of your choice
- 2 tablespoons Capizzano© Medium Intensity Extra Virgin Olive Oil
- 1/4 cup shredded unsweetened coconut

Instructions:

1. In a large mixing bowl, combine the coarsely ground almonds, sea salt, dried fruit, mini chocolate chips, unsweetened coconut and sunflower seeds. Mix well.

2. Mix together the honey, nut butter, and olive oil in a separate bowl.

3. Combine the wet ingredients into the dry ingredients; Mix into a dough like consistency, with hands. Roll into ping pong size balls.

4. Cover and chill for a few hours before serving.

Walnut Green Bean Spread

I've taken this dip to parties, and it gets rave reviews even from teenagers. They've asked for me to bring it again.

Ingredients:

- 1 pound green beans
- Medium sweet onion, thinly sliced (about 1/2 cup)
- 2 tablespoons Picual or Coratina Extra Virgin Olive Oil
- ¼ tsp. Sea Salt to taste
- 1 cup walnuts
- 4 teaspoonslemon juice (I used fresh lemon juice) or 3 tsp. white miso soup
- Add 4 tablespoons Wild Mushroom & Sage Olive Oil in while mixing ingredients in food processor.
- Fresh ground pepper to taste
- Green Scallions and/or Red Bell Peppers, finely chopped for garnish.
- Carrots, Celery or red pepper, sliced thinly to use for dipping

Instructions:

1. Wash & snip green beans.

2. In medium pan low heat, steam the green beans covered in ½ inch of water until tender, about 10 minutes. Drain. Set aside.

3. Slice the onion thinly, should be about ½ cup.

4. Heat the EVOO in a pan over medium heat.

5. Add onions, sauté for 3 minutes.

6. Add sea salt, reduce heat, and cook covered for 5 minutes or until soft.

7. Uncover, raise the heat to medium high cook for 10 minutes until browned, stirring often.

8. Grind walnuts in a food processor.

9. Add the cooked green beans and onions process thoroughly.

10. Add miso or lemon juice, Wild Mushroom & Sage Olive Oil and pepper. Process for a few more seconds, until blended; Should be looking like a hummus spread. If the texture is too thick, add more lemon juice and/or Mushroom & Sage Olive Oil, mix again.

11. Taste and adjust seasoning if needed.

12. Transfer to a glass bowl and drizzle your desired favorite flavor of Extra Virgin Olive Oil on top before serving.

Note:

1. I used Wild Mushroom & Sage Infused Olive Oil. I drizzle a generous amount of Wild Mushroom and Sage Infused Olive Oil on top before serving

2. Cut peppers, celery and/or carrots in thin pieces or use your favorite crackers to dip into this delicious goodness.

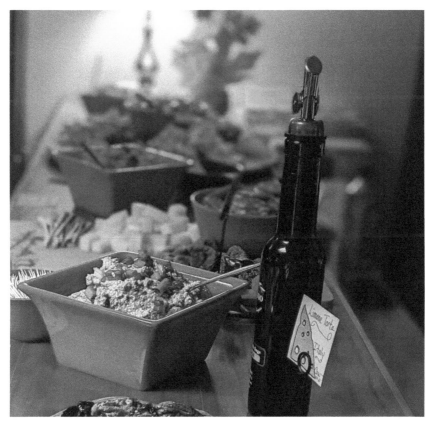

Watermelon Feta with Balsamic Drizzle

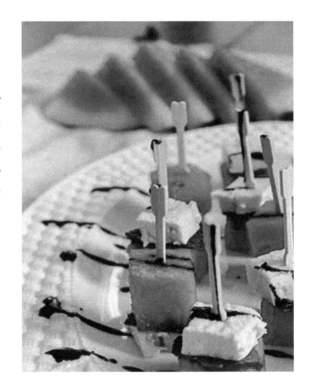

This is a refreshing summer appetizer that combines the sweetness of the watermelon with the saltiness of the feta cheese. The Balsamic drizzle is the icing on the cake.

Ingredients:

- Watermelon cut into squares
- Feta cheese
- Capizzano© Private Reserve 25 Year Aged Balsamic Vinegar

Instructions:

1. Cube ripe watermelon then arrange on plate.

2. take soft feta cheese and mix it up so it is pliable.

3. Put a little of the softened feta chesse on top of the watermelon cube sections.

4. Drizzle Capizzano© Private Reserve 25 Year Aged Balsamic Vinegar over the watermelon and feta cheese.

5. Serve while the watermelon is cold. Use toothpicks for each cube for ease of serving them.

No Bean Hummus

Serves 4

Ingredients:

- 2 zucchinis, peeled and chopped
- ¾ cup raw tahini
- ½ cup fresh lemon juice
- ¼ cup robust intensity Capizzano© Extra Virgin Olive Oil
- 3 cloves garlic, peeled
- 2 ½ teaspoons sea salt
- ½ teaspoon cumin

Instructions:

1. In high-speed blender, combine all the ingredients and blend until thick and smooth.

2. Serve with fresh baked bread, whole grain crackers, raw carrot, cucumber, zucchini or celery slices.

Options:

Garlic or Basil Infused Olive Oils taste great in this hummus too.

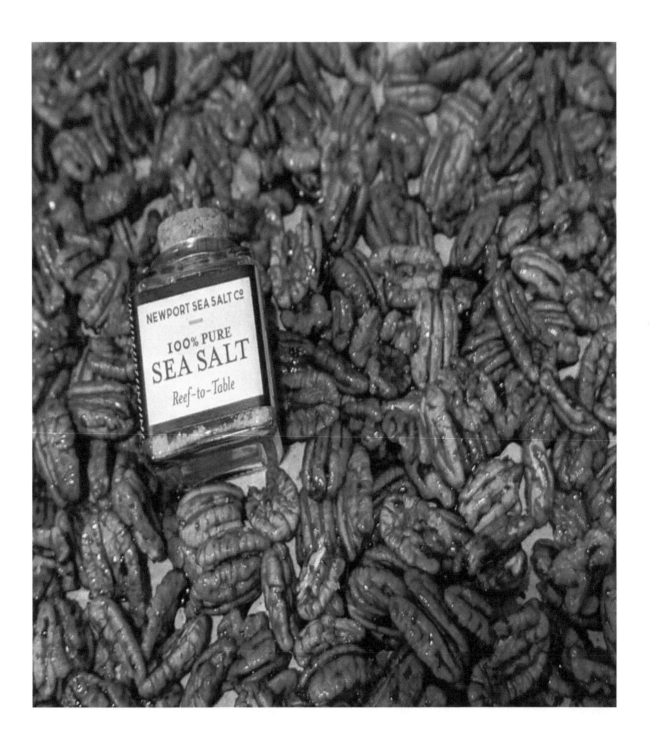

Roasted Maple Pecans

We always add these to our charcuterie board events.
A huge success with cheeses and fruit.

Ingredients:

- 2 cups of Pecans, whole
- 1/2 cup Maple Aged Balsamic Vinegar
- ½ teaspoon of Sea Salt

Instructions:

1. Heat oven to 375 degrees F.

2. In bowl put the pecans, drizzle the Maple Aged Balsamic Vinegar over the pecans, coating them generously.

3. Add a teaspoon of sea salt and toss to cover the pecans with balsamic and sea salt.

4. Place parchment paper on a shallow, large cookie pan.

5. Spread pecans out evenly.

6. Put in oven for about 6 minutes, remove and toss them on the cookie pan.

7. Put them back in the oven for about 6 minutes more; keeping an eye on them as they can burn easily. They should look golden brown when done.

8. Remove and cool on sheet completely.

9. Put in small bags for treats or serve them in a bowl. Cover any remaining pecans. They can last up to a week.

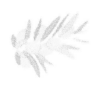

Drinks

Refreshing, Renewing and Replenishing.
A sip says it all with no added sugar.

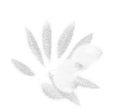

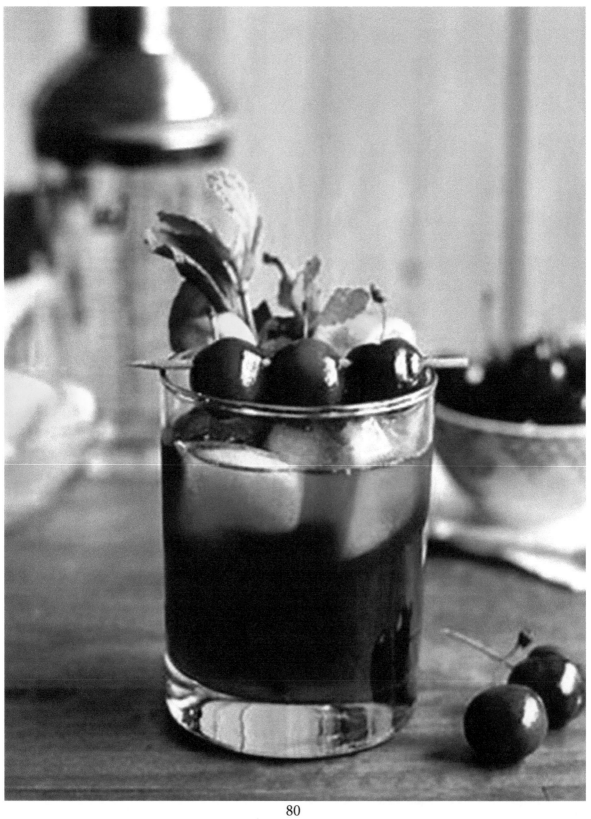

Black Cherry Mint Mocktail

Servings: 4

Ingredients:

- 1 cup pitted fresh or frozen (thawed) black cherries
- ¼ cup fresh mint leaves, plus 4 sprigs for garnish
- 1 ½ ounces of Capizzano© Black Cherry Aged Balsamic Vinegar
- ¼ cup lime juice
- 3 cups cherry-flavored seltzer

Instructions:

1. Put cherries, mint leaves and Black Cherry Aged Balsamic Vinegar in a blender and blend slowly- pulsing several times until chunky smooth.

2. Stir in lime juice.

3. Pour mixture in tall glasses then fill the glasses with ice.

4. Top with seltzer.

5. Garnish with mint sprigs and a couple cherries on a toothpick.

Mango Smoothie

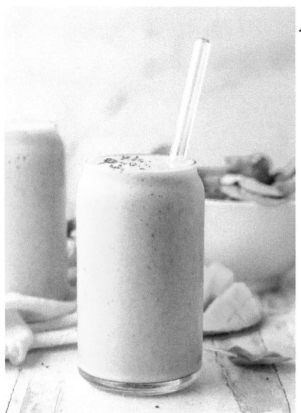

The Persian Lime Olive Oil adds a great fresh lime flavor to complement the coconut water. It is a great way to get your healthy fats in a smoothie.

Picture credit from *Natural Nurturer*

Ingredients:

- ½ cup mangos, frozen
- 1 banana, peeled
- 1 orange, naval, peeled and cut into 4 sections
- 2 large handfuls of baby spinach
- 2 tablespoons of chia seeds
- 3 tablespoons of Capizzano© Persian Lime Infused Olive Oil
- 2 small containers (11 ounces each) of coconut water

Instructions:

1. Add ingredients into your high speed blender

2. blend until completely smooth.

3. Enjoy.

Balsamic Beverage

Enjoy this refreshing drink without any added sugar.

Ingredients:

- 7 ounces of cold water or sparkling water
- 1 ounce of your favorite Aged Balsamic Vinegar flavor
- Ice crushed or cubes.

Instructions:

1. Put the aged balsamic vinegar in a glass.

2. Add some ice and pour the cold water or sparkling water over; stir well.

3. Garnish with lime, lemon, strawberry or raspberry to serve.

4. To make this into a cocktail, add your favorite spirits.

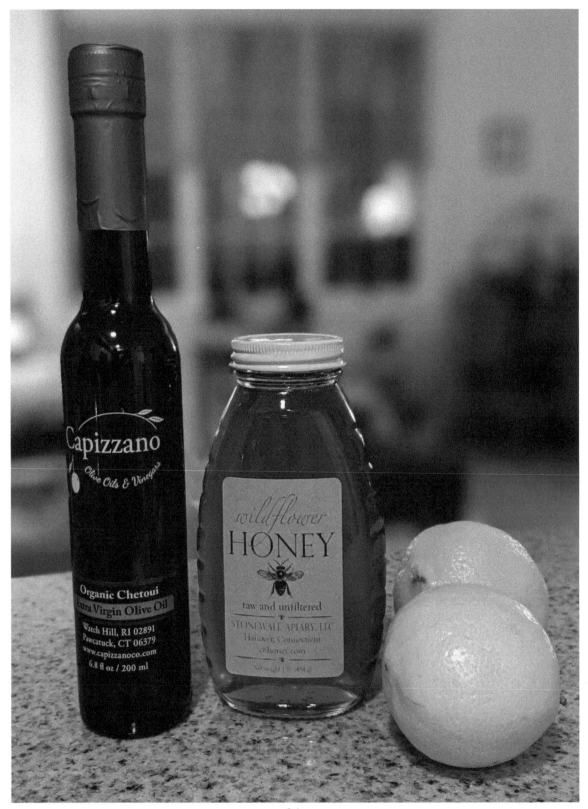

Your Morning Drink

EVOO, Lemon, Honey, Water
To your health!

Ingredients:

2 ounce warm water

1 teaspoon local raw honey

½ fresh lemon, squeezed

2 tablespoons High Phenol "robust intensity" Extra Virgin Olive Oil (EVOO)

Instructions:

1. Mix the warm water and honey together first.

2. Add the lemon juice and EVOO, mix well. Drink immediately.

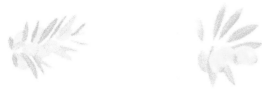

Salsa

Salsas are wonderful to complement any meal. The cranberry orange is refreshing and is great with a charcuterie board for the holidays or with meats. The avocado cilantro tomato salsa is delicious with beans, fish or as a side dish to tacos.

Cranberry Orange 88

Avocado Cilantro Tomato 89

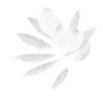
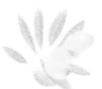

Cranberry Orange Salsa

This is delicious with a charcuterie board complementing gourmet cheeses and as a side dish with poultry. The Cranberry Pear Balsamic Vinegar gives it a crisp clean flavor.

Ingredients:

- 12 ounces fresh or frozen cranberries
- 1/2 cup pure maple syrup
- Zest of 1 medium orange
- Juice of 1 medium orange
- 3 ounces of water
- 2 ounces Cranberry Pear Balsamic Vinegar

Instructions:

1. Place the cranberries in a colander and rinse with cold water. Discard any shriveled or damaged cranberries.

2. In a medium saucepan, combine the cranberries, maple syrup, orange zest, orange juice, and water.

3. Bring to a boil over medium-high heat, then lower the heat to low and simmer, stirring occasionally, until the cranberries have broken down and thickened into a compote, about 20 minutes. The sauce will continue to thicken as it cools.

4. Remove the cranberry sauce from the heat.

5. Cool completely before stirring in the Cranberry Pear Balsamic Vinegar.

6. Transfer to a bowl to chill in the refrigerator.

Avocado Tomato Salsa

Ingredients:

- Avocado, diced
- Tomato, cubed
- Cilantro, snipped
- Onion, minced
- ½ of a small jalepeno pepper, finely diced
- Capizzano© Medium Intensity Extra Virgin Olive Oil
- Juice of a ½ lemon
- Lemon Zest of ½ of a lemon
- Sea Salt

Instructions:

1. Put all ingredients in a bowl.

2. Whisk together the Extra Virgin Olive Oil, lemon juice, lemon zest and sea salt.

3. Pour the olive oil mixture over the ingredients. Fold in gently to coat everything.

4. Let it stand for 15 minutes before serving.

5. Serve with fresh baked bread, corn chips or on top of fish.
   Enjoy the fresh clean flavors!

The Chemistry and Science Behind Olive Oil.

OLEIC ACID

The major fatty acid in olive oil is triacylglycerol, a monounsaturated omega-9 fatty acid which makes up 55 to 85% of the extra virgin olive oil. Higher oleic acid content translates into increase durability and shelf life with greater resistance to oxidation. Extra virgin olive oil is generally higher in oleic acid than other vegetable fats.

FFA (FREE FATTY ACID)

A low FFA is desirable. Free fatty acid speaks to the condition of the fruit at the time of crush. Higher FFA values are indicative of poor-quality fruit such as damaged, overripe, insect infestation, high temperatures during extraction or too much time between harvest and crush.

PEROXIDE VALUE

The primary measurement for rancidity in oil. A very low peroxide value is desirable. Peroxides are formed when oils are exposed to oxygen causing defective flavors and odors. Higher values are indicative of poor quality and/or storage conditions.

PHENOLS

The healthful antioxidant substances in olive oil which aid in slowing down the natural oxidative processes. Phenolic content decreases over time or when exposed to heat, oxygen or light and is an indicator of freshness. Phenols in extra virgin olive oil relate to peppery bitterness and other desirable flavor characteristics. Consuming fresh, well-made olive oil with high phenol content is crucial when looking to obtain the maximum health benefit commonly associated with extra virgin olive oil.

DAG (DIACYLGLYCEROLS)

Low values can indicate oxidized oil & sensory defects. A useful indicator of fruit quality and acts as a snapshot of olive oil freshness.

About the Author

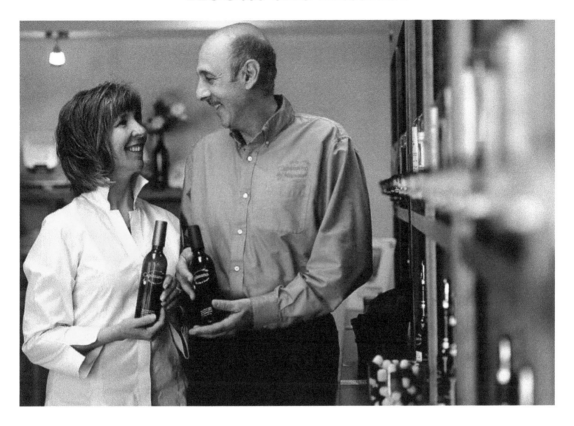

As an experienced health professional in physical therapy and cardiac rehabilitation, **Suzanne Capizzano** knows well the specific benefits of the Mediterranean Lifestyle by choosing high-quality extra virgin olive oils, legumes, vegetables, and fish. She enjoys preparing simple healthy meals with color, texture, and flavor.

For ten years, Suzanne taught a course on a specialized, balanced program that incorporated a medical qigong form called Daoyin Yangsheng Gong. She received her 3rd Duan for Qigong from the Beijing Sports University in March of 2011. She also was a board examiner for the Malcolm Baldrige Recognition Award for a non-profit organization called Quality Council that served NH and VT. Suzanne has enjoyed holding degrees in Physical Therapy, Patient Advocacy, and Workforce Development & Education over the past 25 years. It has been a joy to be of service to many.

Come and visit our Store.
Capizzano Olive Oils & Vinegars
5 Coggswell St,
Pawcatuck, CT 06379

https://CapizzanoCo.com

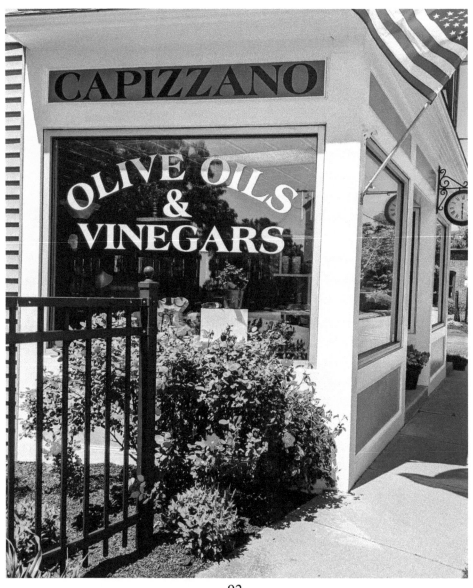

CPSIA information can be obtained
at www.ICGtesting.com
Printed in the USA
BVHW021359031021
618020BV00001B/7